GOUT DIET
COOKBOOK
FOR BEGINNERS

NOURISHING, LOW-PURINE RECIPES TO SUPPORT URIC ACID REGULATION, MINIMIZE JOINT PAIN, AND ENHANCE OVERALL WELLBEING

Ellen A. Milton

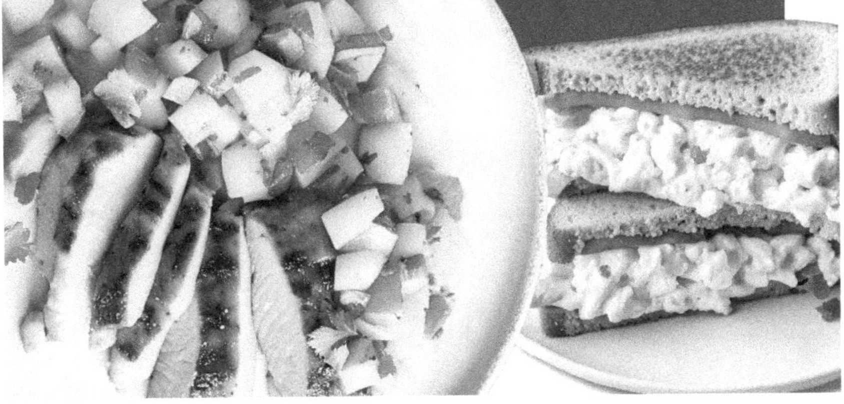

Table Of Content

Introduction

Gout is a disorder that may not get as much attention as other health conditions, but for those who suffer from it, it may be extremely painful. As a newcomer to the gout community, I'm sure you're all too acquainted with the sudden, acute joint pain that may strike without warning. The swelling, redness, and agony are enough to make anybody desire to seek relief.

The good news is that your diet is very important in treating gout, and this cookbook will help you every step of the way. Over the following several chapters, we'll delve in-depth on gout, what causes it, and how the foods you eat may help you avoid painful flare-ups. More significantly, you'll find a delicious collection of low-purine meals that not only feed your body but also promote good uric acid control.

Whether you're new to the gout diet or want to increase your list of gout-friendly foods, this book has you covered. From filling breakfasts to flavor-packed lunches and dinners, as well as quick snacks, guilt-free desserts, and hydrating beverages, each meal has been meticulously developed to help you manage your gout and feel your best.

And don't forget there is a 2-week meal plan, which is a useful tool for getting started and eliminating the guesswork from meal planning. You'll also discover long-term success ideas, like incorporating exercise and managing symptoms, to help you maintain a healthy lifestyle.

Gout may be difficult to manage, but with the correct information and tools, you can regain control of your health and begin enjoying life to its fullest. So, let's dive in and start cooking! Your joints will thank you.

Chapter 1

Understanding Gout

I'm thrilled to begin the first chapter of our Gout Diet Cookbook and help you better understand this often misunderstood ailment. As we engage on this journey together, let us begin by answering some basic questions regarding gout.

What is gout?

Gout is a kind of inflammatory arthritis caused by an excessive accumulation of uric acid in the body. Uric acid is a waste product that the kidneys generally filter out and excreted via urine. However, if the body creates too much uric acid or the kidneys are unable to adequately eliminate it, the extra uric acid may crystallize and accumulate in the joints, causing painful and debilitating symptoms of gout.

1. Uric Acid Buildup: The primary cause of gout is a buildup of uric acid in the body. Uric acid is a natural result of the breakdown of purines, which are contained in many foods we eat. When there is too much uric acid, it may create sharp, needle-like crystals that accumulate in the joints, mainly the big toe, but also in the ankles, heels, knees, and other extremities.

2. Joint Inflammation: The presence of these uric acid crystals causes an inflammatory reaction from the immune system. This causes redness, swelling, stiffness, and severe pain in the afflicted joint. The inflammation may be so acute that even the slightest touch or movement of the joint can be painful.

3. Recurring Attacks: Gout is distinguished by sudden and recurring attacks of joint pain and inflammation. These "flare-ups" might linger for days, if not weeks, before subsiding and returning at a later period. The frequency and intensity of these attacks might vary significantly from person to person.

Understanding the causes behind gout is critical for properly addressing the illness. Individuals with gout may enhance their overall quality of life by addressing the core causes and circumstances that lead to uric acid accumulation.

Causes and symptoms of gout

Gout may be caused by a number of major variables, including:

1. Diet: Consuming foods high in purines, such as red meat, seafood, and some forms of alcohol, will raise uric acid levels. The purines in these meals are degraded into uric acid, which may subsequently build in the body.

2. Genetics: Some people are predisposed to creating high amounts of uric acid or having reduced renal function, which increases their risk of getting gout.

3. Obesity and Metabolic Syndrome: Excess weight, particularly around the waist, raises the risk of gout. Metabolic syndrome, a condition characterized by high blood pressure, excessive blood sugar, and abnormal cholesterol levels, may also lead to gout.

4. Dehydration: Not drinking enough water may cause a buildup of uric acid in the body because the kidneys are unable to adequately wash it out.

5. Certain medications: Some medications, such as diuretics and immunosuppressants, may raise uric acid levels or hinder the kidneys' capacity to eliminate it from the body.

The major sign of gout is acute, intense joint pain, usually in the big toe, although it may also affect the ankles, knees and elbows. The damaged joint may become red, inflamed, and very sensitive to touch, making even little pressure uncomfortable.

In addition to acute joint pain, gout may cause the following symptoms:

1. Inflammation: Uric acid crystals that accumulate in the joints may produce severe inflammation, including swelling, redness, and a burning feeling.

2. Limited Range of Motion: The inflammation and discomfort in the afflicted joint might make it difficult to move, reducing the individual's range of motion.

3. Fever: In rare situations, the body may respond to the presence of uric acid crystals by producing a fever, worsening gout symptoms.

4. Tophi: As uric acid accumulates over time, it may develop hard, lumpy deposits known as tophi, which can appear as visible lumps under the skin and cause further discomfort and stiffness.

Understanding the causes and symptoms of gout is critical for properly treating the disease and avoiding complications. Individuals may take proactive actions to treat gout and enhance their overall health and well-being by knowing the factors that lead to its development and being aware of the common signs and symptoms.

How diet impacts gout

As a beginner, you should comprehend how your food may have a considerable influence on gout treatment.

1. Purine Content: Consuming purine-rich foods is the most important dietary element in treating gout. Purines are chemical molecules that, when broken down, may cause the body to produce more uric acid. Limiting your consumption of purine-rich foods may help manage your uric acid levels and lower your risk of gout flare-ups.

2. Nutrient Balance: In addition to limiting purine consumption, a well-balanced, nutrient-dense diet is essential for gout treatment. Getting adequate vitamins, minerals, and antioxidants may assist improve joint health and minimize inflammation.

3. Hydration: Proper water is required to remove excess uric acid from the body. Drink lots of water throughout the day, since dehydration may lead to uric acid accumulation and raise the risk of gout attacks.

4. Dietary Patterns: Research has indicated that certain dietary patterns may help with gout control. The Mediterranean diet, which emphasizes the intake of fruits and vegetables, whole grains, and healthy fats, has been linked to a decreased incidence of gout flare-ups.

5. Individualized Approach: It's worth noting that the effect of nutrition on gout varies from person to person. While some foods and dietary patterns are generally suggested, it's critical to collaborate with your healthcare physician or a registered dietitian to create a personalized dietary plan that considers your unique requirements, food preferences, and other health issues.

Understanding how nutrition affects gout and implementing the concepts of a low-purine, nutrient-dense diet may help you manage your gout symptoms and improve your overall health. Remember that a holistic approach to gout management, which includes dietary changes, sufficient hydration, and regular physical exercise, will help you get the greatest outcomes.

Chapter 2

Gout-Friendly Ingredients

Okay, let's get into the basics of a gout-friendly diet.

Purines are naturally occurring chemicals that the body converts into uric acid. When uric acid levels get too high, painful crystals form, causing gout flare-ups. By avoiding high-purine meals, you may help regulate your uric acid levels and reduce your risk of gout attacks.

List of low-purine foods

When it comes to controlling gout, it's critical to watch what you eat. Fortunately, there are many tasty and healthy alternatives that are low in purines, which may contribute to the accumulation of uric acid in the body and cause gout flare-ups.

1. Fruits: Fruits are a great option for individuals on a gout diet. Fruits with low purine levels include cherries, berries (blueberries, raspberries, and strawberries), citrus fruits (oranges, grapefruits, lemons, and limes), and apples. These fruits are not only low in purines, but they also include important antioxidants, vitamins, and fiber that may benefit general health.

2. Vegetables: Including a range of low-purine veggies in your diet is an excellent approach to fuel your body while keeping gout under control. Leafy greens (spinach, kale, and arugula), cruciferous vegetables (broccoli, cauliflower, Brussels sprouts), bell peppers, zucchini, and eggplant are also good choices. These veggies are high in important vitamins, minerals, and fiber, making them a key component of a gout-friendly diet.

3. Whole Grains: Whole grains, such as brown rice, quinoa, oats, and whole wheat bread, are low in purines and may offer complex carbs, fiber, and other healthy nutrients. Incorporating these grains into your diet will help you feel full and satisfied while avoiding possible triggers like refined or high-purine grains.

4. Lean Proteins: When choosing protein sources, look for those with low purine levels. Fish (especially salmon, trout, and cod), chicken, turkey, and legumes (such as lentils, chickpeas, and black beans) are all excellent options. These protein-rich foods may be added to a number of gout-friendly recipes without significantly boosting your purine consumption.

5. Dairy Products: A gout-friendly diet may contain low-fat or non-fat milk, yogurt, and cheese. These foods are often low in purines and may supply calcium, protein, and other essential nutrients. However, it is vital to take them in moderation, since high-fat dairy products may not be beneficial for gout.

6. Healthy Fats: Including healthy fats in your diet, such as avocados, nuts, seeds, and olive oil, may help you manage your gout. These fats provide important fatty acids and may assist maintain general health without increasing uric acid levels.

7. Herbs and Spices: Herbs and spices are an excellent method to enhance the taste of your meals without raising the purine level. Garlic, ginger, turmeric, rosemary, and basil are examples of herbs and spices with low purine content. These tasty additives may improve the taste of your meals while also giving health advantages.

Remember that the key to a gout-friendly diet is to eat foods that are low in purines, rich in nutrients, and may promote general health and well-being. By including these low-purine foods into your meals and snacks, you may help control your gout symptoms and lower your risk of future flare-ups.

List of High-Purine Foods and Substitutions

As someone with gout disorder, it's critical to recognize which foods are rich in purines and should be restricted or avoided, as well as appropriate substitutes.

1. Red Meat: Red meat, such as beef, lamb, and pog, is rich in purines and should be avoided.

- **Substitutions:** Choose lean protein sources such as chicken, turkey, fish, and lentils. Grilled chicken breast, baked salmon, and lentil-based recipes are ideal low-purine substitutes.

2. Seafood: Many forms of seafood, such as anchovies, sardines, mussels, scallops, and mackerel, have high levels of purines and should be ingested in moderation.

- **Substitutions:** Choose low-purine fish such as cod, flounder, and tilapia. You may also replace shrimp with canned tuna or grilled tofu.

3. Organ Meats: Organ meats, including liver, kidneys, and sweetbreads, are particularly rich in purines and should be avoided.

- **Substitutions:** Choose lean cuts of muscle meat or plant-based protein sources such as quinoa, tempeh, or edamame.

4. Yeast products: Foods containing yeast, such as bread, beer, and other fermented products, are rich in purines and should be restricted or avoided.

- **Substitutions:** Use yeast-free substitutes such as gluten-free bread, rice cakes, or unsweetened sparkling water.

5. Legumes: While legumes such as beans, lentils, and peas are typically nutritious, they are also rich in purines and should be taken in moderation.

- **Substitutions:** Choose low-purine veggies such as carrots, cucumbers, leafy greens, and bell peppers.

6. Alcohol: Alcoholic drinks, especially beer and liquor, may considerably raise uric acid levels and cause gout attacks.

- **Substitutions:** If you decide to drink, pick lower-purine choices such as wine or distilled spirits in moderation.

Remember that everyone's body reacts differently to particular meals, so pay attention to how yours does and find your own triggers. With a little trial and error, you can figure out which gout-friendly diet works best for you.

Chapter 3

Getting Started with Your Gout Diet

Congratulations for taking the first step in managing gout with a healthy diet! In this chapter, we'll show you how to organize your kitchen, go grocery shopping, plan your meals, and use efficient cooking methods to support your gout-friendly lifestyle.

Setting up your kitchen for success

As you begin on your gout-friendly diet journey, it is critical to prepare your kitchen for success. Creating a supportive atmosphere for your dietary adjustments may make all the difference in sticking to your plan and reaching your health objectives.

Here are some recommendations for making your kitchen gout-friendly:

1. Purge your pantry and refrigerator: The first step is to thoroughly examine the contents of your kitchen and eliminate any high-purine items that might cause gout flare-ups. This includes red meat, organ meats, purine-rich fish (such as sardines, anchovies, and mackerel), alcoholic beverages, and sugary drinks. Replace them with low-purine options such as chicken, turkey, eggs, dairy, whole grains, fruits, and vegetables.

2. Stock up on key low-purine ingredients: To make meal preparation easier, stock your pantry and refrigerator with gout-friendly products.

Some must-have products are:

- Whole grains like brown rice, quinoa, oats, and barley.
- Legumes like lentils, chickpeas, black beans, and kidney beans.
- Leafy greens like spinach, kale, arugula, and Swiss chard.
- Cruciferous vegetables such as broccoli, cauliflower, and Brussels sprouts.
- Berries like blueberries, strawberries, and raspberries.
- Citrus fruits such as oranges, lemons, and limes.
- Healthy fats like olive oil, avocado, almonds, and seeds.
- Herbs and spices such as garlic, ginger, turmeric, rosemary, and basil

3. Buy gout-friendly kitchen tools: Having the proper equipment may make meal preparation simpler and more effective. Consider include the following things in your culinary arsenal:

- Premium chef's knife and cutting board for precision vegetable and fruit preparation.
- Slow cooker or instant pot for hands-free cooking of stews, soups, and bean meals.
- Blender or food processor for creating smoothies, dips, and nut butters.
- Spiralizer for making zucchini noodles and other plant-based pasta alternatives
- A steamer basket or pot for delicately cooking vegetables.

4. Organize your workspace: Decluttering and arranging your kitchen will help you remain focused and productive while making gout-friendly meals. Set aside special locations for your low-purine supplies, cooking tools, and meal prep surfaces. This allows you to easily find the goods you need while maintaining a clean, streamlined work environment.

Setting up your kitchen for success can help you create a gout-friendly atmosphere that supports your health and wellness objectives. Remember, the more prepared and organized you are, the simpler it will be to follow a low-purine diet and successfully manage your gout symptoms.

Grocery shopping tips for a gout diet

Grocery shopping might be intimidating for someone who is new to managing their gout via diet. However, with a little forethought and know-how, it may become a simple and powerful component of your new gout-friendly lifestyle. Allow us to provide some useful suggestions for making your supermarket visits a breeze.

1. Make a Plan: Before going to the shop, evaluate the low-purine meals suggested in this cookbook or elsewhere. Make a list of the items you'll need for the dishes you want to test in the coming weeks. This can help you remain focused and avoid making impulsive purchases that might derail your diet.

2. Read Labels Carefully: When choosing packaged goods, pay particular attention to the nutrition labels. Pay close attention to the purine content, sodium levels, and any other components that might cause gout flare-ups. Choose low-purine, low-sodium.

3. Familiarize Yourself with Purine-Rich Foods: Memorize the list of high-purine foods to avoid, which includes red meat, seafood, sugary beverages, and some kinds of beans and lentils. This will make it easy to identify and avoid certain goods when traveling the shopping aisles.

4. Look for Substitutes: If you come across a recipe that requires a high-purine component, take a time to find an appropriate low-purine substitute. For example, substitute beef for turkey, low-fat dairy for full-fat, and quinoa or brown rice instead of high-purine grains.

5. Buy in Bulk: Many of the essential foods in a gout-friendly diet, including fruits, vegetables, nuts, and whole grains, may be bought in bulk. This not only saves you money, but also guarantees that you always have these nutritious alternatives available for meal preparation.

6. Explore the Produce department: The bright produce department might help you combat gout. Load up on a range of colorful fruits and vegetables that are high in nutrients and low in purines. Don't be hesitant to explore new, gout-friendly products you haven't seen before.

7. Embrace Frozen Options: Frozen fruits and veggies may be just as healthy as fresh ones, plus they have a longer shelf life. Stock up on frozen fruit and leafy vegetables to make meal prep easier.

8. Hydrate with Water: Fill your cart with lots of bottled or filtered water. As we discussed, staying hydrated is essential for eliminating uric acid and avoiding gout flare-ups.

9. Shop the Perimeter: As a general guideline, shop the grocery store's outside aisles for the freshest, most healthful items. Avoid spending too much time in the middle aisles, which are usually filled with processed, high-purine foods.

By following these gout-friendly grocery shopping suggestions, you'll be well on your way to filling your kitchen with the vital elements for gout treatment. Remember that consistency is important, so make this a regular part of your routine. Happy (and healthy) shopping!

Meal planning strategies

Meal planning is an essential part of a successful gout control diet. Planning your meals ahead of time ensures that you have a consistent supply of gout-friendly foods on hand, making it simpler to adhere to your diet. Here are some helpful meal planning methods to get you started:

1. Weekly Meal Prep: Set aside time, maybe over the weekend, to prepare and divide up your meals for the next week. This might include cutting veggies, preparing grains, pre-portioning protein, and putting together salads or bowls. Having these ingredients on hand makes it much easier to prepare a fast, gout-friendly meal on the busiest weekdays.

2. Make a Meal Calendar: Spend some time planning out your meals for the week, or possibly the month. This might assist you ensure that you're eating a range of low-purine meals and balancing your nutritional needs. When preparing your meal calendar, consider your schedule, available cooking time, and any social activities or dining out plan.

3. Batch Cooking: Set aside one or two days each week to create big amounts of gout-friendly foods including soups, stews, and casseroles. These may then be portioned and kept in the refrigerator or freezer for easy reheating on busy days.

4. Meal Kits and Delivery Services: If you find meal planning and preparation difficult, try using a meal kit or meal delivery service that provides gout-friendly alternatives. These services provide pre-portioned ingredients and simple recipes, taking the guesswork out of meal planning and preparation.

5. Maintain a Gout-Friendly Pantry and Fridge: Stock your kitchen with low-purine foods. This will make it simpler to swiftly prepare meals or snacks that are suitable for your gout control diet.

6. Involve the Whole Family: If you live with others, try including them in the meal planning and preparation process. This may help guarantee that everyone in the home supports the gout-friendly diet and makes it simpler to keep to the plan.

7. Weekend Meal Planning: While it is essential to follow a gout-friendly diet throughout the week, weekends may provide extra problems. Meal planning over the weekend might help you remain on track and avoid potential temptations.

Remember that the key to effective meal planning for a gout-friendly diet is identifying solutions that work best for your lifestyle and tastes. Experiment with several ways to see what makes you feel powerful and in charge of your gout treatment.

Cooking techniques for a gout-friendly diet

When it comes to controlling gout with food, how you cook your meals may make a big impact. Certain cooking techniques may help retain the nutritional content of your foods while reducing their influence on your uric acid levels. Let's look at some gout-friendly cooking strategies that can help you in the kitchen:

1. Steaming: Steaming is a wonderful approach for preparing gout-friendly meals. It keeps the natural tastes, minerals, and texture of vegetables, grains, and lean proteins without subjecting them to high temperatures, which might promote the development of uric acid. Steaming is a gentle technique to prepare vegetables like asparagus, broccoli, cauliflower, and fish, preserving their nutritious characteristics.

2. Sautéing: When done correctly, sautéing may be an excellent method of preparing low-purine foods for your gout diet. Choose healthy oils, such as olive or avocado oil, and sauté your items over medium heat. This approach enhances the natural tastes of the food without exposing it to extended high heat, which might cause purine breakdown.

3. Baking: Baking is a flexible culinary method that works well with many gout-friendly foods. From roasted vegetables to baked fish or lean meats, this approach delivers rich, caramelized tastes without the intense heat associated with frying. Consider using herbs, spices, and lemon juice instead of high-purine condiments.

4. Poaching: Poaching is a gentle cooking technique that involves immersing your items in a simmering liquid, such as broth or water. This approach works especially well with delicate proteins like fish and eggs, enabling them to simmer without drying out or losing nutritional content. Poaching is an effective method for preparing meals that are low in purines.

5. Slow Cooking: Slow cooking, whether in a slow cooker or a low-temperature oven, is an excellent way to prepare gout-friendly dishes. This gentle, lengthy cooking procedure breaks down harder components, such as lean meats and legumes, while maintaining their nutritional value. Slow cooking enables the flavors to combine, yielding highly enjoyable and gout-friendly foods.

6. Grilling: Grilling may be a healthy and delectable method to prepare gout-friendly dishes, as long as you pay attention to the cooking temperature and time. Choose lean proteins like chicken, fish, or tofu and serve with grilled veggies like asparagus, bell peppers, or zucchini. Avoid charring or burning food, since this might cause the development of uric acid-raising chemicals.

By adopting these gout-friendly cooking methods into your daily routine, you'll be able to prepare tasty, nutritious meals that promote overall health and help manage your gout symptoms. Remember, the idea is to explore, discover what works best for you, and enjoy the process of creating nutritious meals.

Chapter 4

70+ Low-Purine Recipe

Breakfast Recipes

---

1. Muesli with Almond Milk

Total Time: 10 minutes | Serves 5

Ingredients

- 2 cups rolled oats
- 1/2 cup sliced almonds
- 1/4 cup raisins
- 1/4 cup dried cranberries
- 1 teaspoon ground cinnamon
- 2 cups unsweetened almond milk

Instructions

1. In a large bowl, combine the rolled oats, sliced almonds, raisins, dried cranberries, and ground cinnamon.
2. Pour the almond milk over the muesli mixture and stir to combine.
3. Serve chilled or at room temperature.

Per serving: - Calories: 221 - Fiber: 5g - Carbs: 33g - Fat: 8g - Protein: 6g - Sugar: 12g

2. Avocado Toast with Tomato Slices

Total Time: 15 minutes | Serves 5

Ingredients

- 10 slices whole-grain bread
- 2 ripe avocados, mashed
- 1 teaspoon lemon juice
- 1/2 teaspoon salt
- 5 tomatoes, sliced

Instructions

1. Toast the whole-grain bread.
2. In a small bowl, mash the avocados with lemon juice and salt.
3. Spread the mashed avocado mixture evenly on the toasted bread.
4. Top each slice with 2-3 tomato slices.

Per serving: - Calories: 258 - Fiber: 8g - Carbs: 32g - Fat: 12g - Protein: 7g - Sugar: 5g

3. Breakfast Burrito with Black Beans

Total Time: 20 minutes | Serves 5

Ingredients

- 5 whole-wheat tortillas
- 1 (15 oz) can black beans (drained and rinsed)
- 1 cup diced bell peppers
- 1/2 cup diced onion
- 2 eggs, scrambled
- 1/4 cup shredded cheddar cheese

Instructions

1. In a skillet, sauté the diced bell peppers and onions until soft.
2. Add the black beans and warm through.
3. In a different pan, scramble the eggs.
4. Lay the tortillas flat and evenly distribute the black bean mixture, scrambled eggs, and shredded cheese.
5. Fold the tortilla into a burrito and serve.

Per serving: - Calories: 320 - Fiber: 10g - Carbs: 42g - Fat: 10g - Protein: 16g - Sugar: 3g

4. Scrambled Eggs with Spinach

Total Time: 15 minutes | Serves 5

Ingredients

- 10 eggs
- 2 cups fresh spinach, chopped
- 2 tablespoons milk
- 1/4 teaspoon salt
- 1/4 teaspoon black pepper

Instructions

1. In a medium bowl, whisk the eggs, milk, salt, and pepper.
2. In a skillet over medium heat, sauté the chopped spinach until wilted.
3. Pour the egg mixture into the skillet and scramble until cooked through.

Per serving: - Calories: 177 - Fiber: 1g - Carbs: 3g - Fat: 11g - Protein: 16g - Sugar: 1g

5. Whole Grain Pancakes with Maple Syrup

Total Time: 30 minutes | Serves 5

Ingredients

- 1 cup whole-wheat flour
- 1 teaspoon baking powder
- 1/4 teaspoon salt
- 1 cup unsweetened almond milk
- 1 egg
- 1 tablespoon honey
- 1 tablespoon melted coconut oil
- 1/4 cup 100% pure maple syrup

Instructions

1. In a large bowl, whisk together the whole-wheat flour, baking powder, and salt.
2. In a different bowl, whisk the almond milk, egg, honey, and melted coconut oil.
3. Pour the wet ingredients into the dry ingredients and stir until just combined (carefull, do not overmix).
4. Heat a non-stick skillet or griddle over medium heat. Scoop 1/4 cup of batter per pancake and cook for 2-3 minutes per side, or until golden brown.
5. Serve the pancakes warm, drizzled with maple syrup.

Per serving: - Calories: 270 - Fiber: 4g - Carbs: 40g - Fat: 10g - Protein: 8g - Sugar: 16g

6. Green Smoothie with Kale and Pineapple

Total Time: 10 minutes | Serves 3

Ingredients

- 2 cups kale, chopped
- 1 cup pineapple chunks
- 1 cup unsweetened almond milk
- 1 banana, frozen
- 1 tablespoon honey (optional)

Instructions

1. Add all the ingredients to a high-speed blender.
2. Blend until smooth and creamy.
3. Pour the smoothie into glasses and enjoy.

Per serving: - Calories: 150 - Fiber: 4g - Carbs: 30g - Fats: 2g - Protein: 4g - Sugar: 20g

7. Banana Walnut Smoothie

Total Time: 10 minutes | Serves 3

Ingredients

- 2 bananas, frozen
- 1 cup unsweetened almond milk
- 1/4 cup walnuts
- 1 tablespoon honey (optional)
- 1/2 teaspoon cinnamon

Instructions

1. Add all the ingredients to a high-speed blender.
2. Blend until smooth and creamy.
3. Pour the smoothie into glasses and enjoy.

Per serving: - Calories: 190 - Fiber: 4g - Carbs: 28g - Fats: 8g - Protein: 5g - Sugar: 16g

8. Cinnamon Raisin Toast with Ricotta

Total Time: 15 minutes | Serves 3

Ingredients

- 6 slices whole-grain bread
- 1/2 cup ricotta cheese
- 2 tablespoons raisins
- 1 teaspoon ground cinnamon

Instructions

1. Toast the bread until lightly golden.
2. Spread 2 tablespoons of ricotta cheese onto each slice of toast.
3. Sprinkle 1 teaspoon of raisins and a pinch of cinnamon on top of the ricotta.
4. Serve immediately and enjoy.

Per serving: - Calories: 210 - Fiber: 4g - Carbs: 30g - Fats: 8g - Protein: 10g - Sugar: 10g

9. Cottage Cheese with Pineapple

Total Time: 10 minutes | Serves 3

Ingredients

- 1 cup cottage cheese
- 1 cup pineapple chunks
- 1 tablespoon honey (optional)

Instructions

1. Divide the cottage cheese evenly into three bowls.
2. Top each serving with 1/3 cup of pineapple chunks.
3. Drizzle 1 teaspoon of honey over the pineapple (optional).

Per serving: - Calories: 130 - Fiber: 2g - Carbs: 15g - Fats: 5g - Protein: 12g - Sugar: 12g

10. Rice Cake with Hummus and Cucumber

Total Time: 10 minutes | Serves 3

Ingredients

- 6 whole-grain rice cakes
- 1/2 cup hummus
- 1 cucumber, sliced

Instructions

1. Spread 2 tablespoons of hummus evenly on each rice cake.
2. Top with sliced cucumber.
3. Serve immediately and enjoy.

Per serving: - Calories: 150 - Fiber: 4g - Carbs: 20g - Fats: 6g - Protein: 6g - Sugar: 2g

11. Smoked Salmon and Cream Cheese Bagel

Total Time: 20 minutes | Serves 3

Ingredients

- 3 whole-grain bagels, halved
- 6 ounces smoked salmon
- 3 tablespoons cream cheese
- 1 tablespoon capers (optional)
- 1 tablespoon chopped dill (optional)

Instructions

1. Toast the bagel halves until lightly golden.
2. Spread 1 tablespoon of cream cheese on each bagel half.
3. Top with 2 ounces of smoked salmon.
4. Sprinkle with capers and chopped dill (optional).
5. Serve immediately and enjoy.

Per serving: - Calories: 260 - Fiber: 3g - Carbs: 28g - Fats: 12g - Protein: 16g - Sugar: 2g

12. Fruit Salad with Mint

Total Time: 20 minutes | Serves 3

Ingredients

- 1 cup diced pineapple
- 1 cup diced strawberries
- 1 cup diced cantaloupe
- 1/4 cup chopped fresh mint
- 1 tablespoon honey (optional)

Instructions

1. In a large bowl, combine the diced pineapple, strawberries, and cantaloupe.
2. Sprinkle the chopped mint over the fruit.
3. Drizzle the honey over the fruit salad (optional).
4. Toss gently to combine.
5. Serve immediately or chill until ready to serve.

Per serving: - Calories: 100 - Fiber: 3g - Carbs: 24g - Fats: 0g - Protein: 1g - Sugar: 18g

13. Buckwheat Porridge with Cinnamon

Total Time: 30 minutes | Serves 3

Ingredients

- 1 cup buckwheat groats
- 3 cups unsweetened almond milk
- 1 teaspoon ground cinnamon
- 1 tablespoon honey (optional)
- 1/4 cup chopped walnuts (optional)

Instructions

1. In a medium saucepan, combine the buckwheat groats and almond milk.
2. Bring the mixture to a boil, then reduce the heat and simmer for 15-20 minutes, stirring occasionally, until the buckwheat is tender and the porridge has thickened.
3. Remove from heat and stir in the cinnamon.
4. Divide the porridge into three bowls and drizzle with honey and chopped walnuts (optional).

Per serving: - Calories: 280 - Fiber: 6g - Carbs: 37g - Fats: 10g - Protein: 9g - Sugar: 8g

14. Almond Butter Toast with Sliced Apples

Total Time: 15 minutes | Serves 3

Ingredients

- 6 slices whole-grain bread
- 6 tablespoons almond butter
- 1 apple, thinly sliced
- 1 teaspoon ground cinnamon (optional)

Instructions

1. Toast the bread until lightly golden.
2. Spread 1 tablespoon of almond butter on each slice of toast.
3. Top with sliced apples.
4. Sprinkle with ground cinnamon (optional).
5. Serve immediately and enjoy.

Per serving: - Calories: 270 - Fiber: 6g - Carbs: 30g - Fats: 13g - Protein: 10g - Sugar: 8g

15. Tomato Basil Bruschetta

Total Time: 20 minutes | Serves 3

Ingredients

- 6 slices whole-grain baguette or toast
- 1 cup diced tomatoes
- 1/4 cup chopped fresh basil
- 2 tablespoons balsamic glaze
- 1 tablespoon olive oil
- 1 garlic clove, minced
- Salt and pepper to taste

Instructions

1. Preheat your oven to 400°F (200°C).
2. Place the bread slices on a baking sheet and toast in the oven for 5-7 minutes, or until lightly golden.
3. In a small bowl, combine the diced tomatoes, chopped basil, balsamic glaze, olive oil, and minced garlic. Season with salt and pepper.
4. Top the toasted bread slices with the tomato basil mixture.
5. Serve immediately and enjoy.

Per serving: - Calories: 160 - Fiber: 3g - Carbs: 23g - Fats: 6g - Protein: 5g - Sugar: 4g

Lunch Recipes

---

1. Lentil Salad with Cherry Tomatoes

Total Time: 30 minutes | Serves 4

Ingredients

- 1 cup cooked brown lentils
- 1 cup cherry tomatoes, halved
- 1/2 cup diced cucumber
- 1/4 cup crumbled feta cheese
- 2 tablespoons chopped fresh parsley
- 2 tablespoons olive oil
- 1 tablespoon lemon juice
- 1 garlic clove, minced
- 1/4 teaspoon salt
- 1/8 teaspoon black pepper

Instructions

1. In a large bowl, add the cooked lentils, cherry tomatoes, cucumber, feta cheese, and parsley.
2. In a small bowl, whisk together the olive oil, lemon juice, garlic, salt, and black pepper.
3. Pour the dressing over the lentil salad and gently toss to combine.
4. Serve chilled or at room temperature.

Per serving: - Calories: 165 - Fiber: 7g - Carbs: 17g - Fat: 9g - Protein: 8g - Sugar: 3g

2. Grilled Chicken Caesar Salad

Total Time: 30 minutes | Serves 4

Ingredients

- 4 boneless, skinless chicken breasts
- 1 romaine lettuce heart, chopped
- 1/2 cup croutons
- 1/4 cup grated Parmesan cheese
- 2 tablespoons Caesar dressing

Instructions

1. Preheat a grill or a grill pan to medium-high heat.
2. Grill the chicken breasts for 4-6 minutes per side, or until cooked through.
3. Let the chicken rest for 5 minutes, then slice or chop it.
4. In a large salad bowl, combine the chopped romaine, grilled chicken, croutons, and Parmesan cheese.
5. Drizzle the Caesar dressing over the salad and toss gently to coat.

Per serving: - Calories: 235 - Fiber: 2g - Carbs: 8g - Fat: 9g - Protein: 31g - Sugar: 2g

3. Salmon and Asparagus Foil Packets

Total Time: 30 minutes | Serves 4

Ingredients

- 4 (6-ounce) salmon fillets
- 1 pound fresh asparagus, trimmed
- 2 tablespoons olive oil
- 1 lemon, zested and juiced
- 1 garlic clove, minced
- 1/4 teaspoon salt
- 1/8 teaspoon black pepper

Instructions

1. Preheat your oven to 400°F.
2. Cut four 12-inch square pieces of heavy-duty aluminum foil.
3. In the center of each foil piece, place one salmon fillet and a quarter of the asparagus.
4. In a small bowl, whisk together the olive oil, lemon zest, lemon juice, garlic, salt, and pepper.
5. Drizzle the lemon-garlic mixture over the salmon and asparagus.
6. Fold the foil over the salmon and asparagus, and crimp the edges to form a sealed packet.
7. Place the foil packets on a baking sheet and bake for 15-20 minutes, or until the salmon is cooked through and the asparagus is tender.
8. Gently open the foil packets and serve.

Per serving: - Calories: 225 - Fiber: 3g - Carbs: 3g - Fat: 12g - Protein: 25g - Sugar: 1g

4. Eggplant and Tomato Panini

Total Time: 30 minutes | Serves 4

Ingredients

- 1 medium eggplant (sliced into 1/4-inch thick rounds)
- 2 tablespoons olive oil
- 1/2 teaspoon salt
- 1/4 teaspoon black pepper
- 8 slices whole-wheat bread
- 8 slices fresh mozzarella cheese
- 1 cup cherry tomatoes, sliced

Instructions

1. Preheat a panini press or a grill pan to medium-high heat.
2. In a large bowl, toss the eggplant slices with the olive oil, salt, and black pepper.
3. Grill the eggplant slices for 2-3 minutes per side, or until they are softened and lightly charred.
4. Assemble the paninis by layering the grilled eggplant, mozzarella cheese, and sliced cherry tomatoes between the whole-wheat bread slices.
5. Grill the paninis in the panini press or grill pan for 3-4 minutes per side, or until the bread is golden brown and the cheese is melted.
6. Serve!

Per serving: - Calories: 310 - Fiber: 6g - Carbs: 34g - Fat: 15g - Protein: 16g - Sugar: 6g

5. Chickpea and Cucumber Salad

Total Time: 20 minutes | Serves 4

Ingredients

- 1 (15-ounce) can chickpeas (drained and rinsed)
- 1 English cucumber, diced
- 1/4 cup diced red onion
- 2 tablespoons chopped fresh parsley
- 2 tablespoons olive oil
- 1 tablespoon lemon juice
- 1/4 teaspoon salt
- 1/8 teaspoon black pepper

Instructions

1. In a large bowl, add the chickpeas, diced cucumber, red onion, and chopped parsley.
2. In a small bowl, whisk together the olive oil, lemon juice, salt, and black pepper.
3. Pour the dressing over the chickpea and cucumber salad and toss gently to coat.
4. Serve the salad chilled or at room temperature.

Per serving: - Calories: 155 - Fiber: 6g - Carbs: 18g - Fat: 8g - Protein: 5g - Sugar: 3g

6. Turkey and Avocado Wrap

Total Time: 20 minutes | Serves 4

Ingredients

- 4 whole wheat tortillas
- 8 oz sliced turkey breast
- 2 avocados, sliced
- 1 cup baby spinach leaves
- 1/4 cup plain Greek yogurt
- 1 tbsp lemon juice
- Salt and pepper to taste

Instructions

1. Lay the tortillas flat on a clean surface.
2. Evenly distribute the sliced turkey, avocado, and spinach leaves onto the center of each tortilla.
3. In a small bowl, mix the Greek yogurt and lemon juice. Spread this mixture over the fillings.
4. Season with salt and pepper.
5. Fold the bottom of the tortilla up, then fold in the sides and continue rolling tightly.

Per serving: - Calories: 290 - Fiber: 6g - Carbs: 24g - Fat: 15g - Protein: 20g - Sugar: 2g

7. Caprese Salad with Balsamic Glaze

Total Time: 20 minutes | Serves 4

Ingredients

- 8 oz fresh mozzarella cheese, sliced
- 2 large tomatoes, sliced
- 1/4 cup fresh basil leaves
- 2 tbsp balsamic glaze
- 1 tbsp extra-virgin olive oil
- Salt and pepper to taste

Instructions

1. Arrange the mozzarella and tomato slices on a serving platter.
2. Scatter the fresh basil leaves over the top.
3. Drizzle the balsamic glaze and olive oil over the salad.
4. Season with salt and pepper to taste.

Per serving: - Calories: 180 - Fiber: 2g - Carbs: 6g - Fat: 13g - Protein: 12g - Sugar: 4g

8. Roasted Beet and Goat Cheese Salad

Total Time: 50 minutes | Serves 4

Ingredients

- 4 medium beets (peeled and cut into wedges)
- 1 tbsp olive oil
- Salt and pepper to taste
- 5 oz mixed greens
- 2 oz crumbled goat cheese
- 2 tbsp toasted walnuts
- 2 tbsp balsamic vinegar
- 1 tbsp honey

Instructions

1. Preheat your oven to 400°F. Toss the beet wedges with olive oil, salt, and pepper.
2. Roast the beets for 30-35 minutes, or until tender.
3. In a large salad bowl, mix the roasted beets, mixed greens, goat cheese, and toasted walnuts.
4. In a small bowl, whisk together the balsamic vinegar and honey. Drizzle the dressing over the salad.
5. Toss gently to coat.

Per serving: - Calories: 210 - Fiber: 4g - Carbs: 18g - Fat: 13g - Protein: 8g - Sugar: 12g

9. Zucchini Noodles with Pesto

Total Time: 20 minutes | Serves 4

Ingredients

- 3 medium zucchinis (spiralized or julienned)
- 1/2 cup homemade (or store-bought basil pesto)
- 2 tbsp grated Parmesan cheese
- Salt and pepper to taste

Instructions

1. In a large bowl, toss the zucchini noodles with the pesto until well coated.
2. Sprinkle the grated Parmesan cheese over the top.
3. Season with salt and pepper to taste.
4. Serve immediately and enjoy.

Per serving: - Calories: 140 - Fiber: 3g - Carbs: 8g - Fat: 10g - Protein: 5g - Sugar: 3g

10. Spinach and Goat Cheese Stuffed Chicken Breast

Total Time: 50 minutes | Serves 4

Ingredients

- 4 boneless, skinless chicken breasts
- 4 oz crumbled goat cheese
- 1 cup fresh baby spinach, chopped
- 1 tbsp olive oil
- Salt and pepper to taste

Instructions

1. Preheat your oven to 375°F.
2. Use a sharp knife to cut a pocket into the side of each chicken breast.
3. In a small bowl, mix the crumbled goat cheese and chopped spinach.
4. Stuff the cheese-spinach mixture evenly into the pockets of the chicken breasts.
5. Heat the olive oil in a large oven-safe skillet over medium-high heat.
6. Add the stuffed chicken breasts and sear for 2-3 minutes per side.
7. Take the skillet to the oven and bake for 20-25 minutes, or until the chicken is cooked through.
8. Season with salt and pepper to taste.

Per serving: - Calories: 270 - Fiber: 1g - Carbs: 2g - Fat: 12g - Protein: 37g - Sugar: 1g

11. Egg Salad Sandwich on Whole Wheat Bread

Total Time: 30 minutes | Serves 5

Ingredients

- 6 hard-boiled eggs, chopped
- 2 tbsp low-fat mayonnaise
- 1 tbsp Dijon mustard
- 2 tsp lemon juice
- 1/4 cup diced celery
- 2 tbsp diced onion
- 1/4 tsp salt
- 1/8 tsp black pepper
- 10 slices whole wheat bread

Instructions

1. In a medium bowl, add the chopped hard-boiled eggs, mayonnaise, Dijon mustard, lemon juice, celery, onion, salt, and black pepper. Mix well.
2. Divide the egg salad evenly among the 10 slices of whole wheat bread to make 5 sandwiches.

Per serving: - Calories: 240 - Fiber: 4g - Carbs: 30g - Fat: 9g - Protein: 14g - Sugar: 3g

12. Shrimp and Avocado Salad

Total Time: 30 minutes | Serves 5

Ingredients

- 1 lb cooked shrimp (peeled and deveined)
- 2 avocados, diced
- 1/2 cup diced cucumber
- 1/4 cup diced red onion
- 2 tbsp chopped fresh cilantro
- 2 tbsp olive oil
- 1 tbsp lime juice
- 1/4 tsp salt
- 1/8 tsp black pepper

Instructions

1. In a large bowl, combine the cooked shrimp, diced avocados, cucumber, red onion, and chopped cilantro.
2. Drizzle with olive oil and lime juice, then season with salt and black pepper. Gently toss to combine.

Per serving: - Calories: 270 - Fiber: 6g - Carbs: 10g - Fat: 18g - Protein: 20g - Sugar: 2g

13. Greek Salad with Feta Cheese

Total Time: 30 minutes | Serves 5

Ingredients

- 5 cups chopped romaine lettuce
- 1 cup diced cucumber
- 1 cup halved cherry tomatoes
- 1/2 cup diced red onion
- 1/2 cup crumbled feta cheese
- 2 tbsp olive oil
- 1 tbsp red wine vinegar
- 1 tsp dried oregano
- 1/4 tsp salt
- 1/8 tsp black pepper

Instructions

1. In a large salad bowl, combine the chopped romaine lettuce, diced cucumber, halved cherry tomatoes, and diced red onion.
2. Sprinkle the crumbled feta cheese over the top.
3. In a small bowl, whisk together the olive oil, red wine vinegar, dried oregano, salt, and black pepper.
4. Drizzle the dressing over the salad and toss gently to combine.

Per serving: - Calories: 180 - Fiber: 3g - Carbs: 10g - Fat: 14g - Protein: 6g - Sugar: 5g

14. Turkey and Spinach Roll-Ups

Total Time: 20 minutes | Serves 5

Ingredients

- 10 slices deli-style turkey
- 2 cups fresh spinach leaves
- 1/2 avocado, sliced
- 2 tbsp cream cheese, softened
- 1 tbsp lemon juice
- 1/4 tsp salt
- 1/8 tsp black pepper

Instructions

1. In a small bowl, mix the softened cream cheese, lemon juice, salt, and black pepper until well combined.
2. Lay the slices of turkey on a flat surface. Place a few spinach leaves and a couple of avocado slices on each turkey slice.
3. Spread a thin layer of the cream cheese mixture on top of the spinach and avocado.
4. Carefully roll up each turkey slice and secure it with a toothpick.

Per serving: - Calories: 150 - Fiber: 2g - Carbs: 3g - Fat: 9g - Protein: 15g - Sugar: 1g

15. Mushroom Barley Soup

Total Time: 60 minutes | Serves 5

Ingredients

- 1 tbsp olive oil
- 1 cup diced onion
- 8 oz sliced mushrooms
- 2 cloves garlic, minced
- 1 cup uncooked pearl barley
- 4 cups low-sodium vegetable broth
- 2 cups water
- 1 tsp dried thyme
- 1/4 tsp salt
- 1/8 tsp black pepper
- 2 cups chopped spinach

Instructions

1. In a large pot, heat the olive oil over medium heat. Add the diced onion and sauté for 3-4 minutes until translucent.
2. Add the sliced mushrooms and minced garlic. Sauté for an additional 2-3 minutes.
3. Stir in the uncooked pearl barley, vegetable broth, water, dried thyme, salt, and black pepper. Bring the mixture to a boil.
4. Reduce the heat to low, cover, and simmer for 25-30 minutes, or until the barley is tender.
5. Stir in the chopped spinach and cook for an additional 2-3 minutes until the spinach is wilted.

Per serving: - Calories: 220 - Fiber: 6g - Carbs: 38g - Fat: 5g - Protein: 7g - Sugar: 3g

Dinner Recipes

1. Baked Halibut with Asparagus

Total Time: 30 minutes | Serves 2

Ingredients

- 2 (4-ounce) halibut fillets
- 1 lb asparagus, trimmed
- 1 tablespoon olive oil
- 1 clove garlic, minced
- 1 teaspoon lemon juice
- Salt and pepper to taste

Instructions

1. Preheat your oven to 400°F.
2. Place the halibut fillets on a baking sheet lined with parchment paper.
3. In a bowl, toss the asparagus with olive oil, garlic, lemon juice, salt, and pepper.
4. Arrange the asparagus around the halibut fillets.
5. Bake for 15-20 minutes, or until the halibut is cooked through and the asparagus is tender.

Per serving: - Calories: 210 - Fiber: 4g - Carbs: 6g - Fat: 9g - Protein: 28g - Sugar: 2g

2. Lentil and Vegetable Stew

Total Time: 60 minutes | Serves 2

Ingredients

- 1 cup brown lentils, rinsed
- 2 cups low-sodium vegetable broth
- 1 tablespoon olive oil
- 1 onion, diced
- 2 carrots, diced
- 2 celery stalks, diced
- 3 cloves garlic, minced
- 1 teaspoon dried thyme
- 1 teaspoon dried oregano
- Salt and pepper to taste

Instructions

1. In a large pot, combine the lentils and vegetable broth. Bring to a boil, then reduce heat and simmer for 20-25 minutes, or until lentils are tender.
2. In a different skillet, heat the olive oil over medium heat. Add the onion, carrots, celery, and garlic. Sauté for 5-7 minutes, until vegetables are softened.
3. Add the sautéed vegetables, thyme, and oregano to the cooked lentils. Season with salt and pepper to taste.
4. Simmer the stew for an additional 10 minutes to allow the flavors to meld.

Per serving: - Calories: 300 - Fiber: 12g - Carbs: 46g - Fat: 7g - Protein: 16g - Sugar: 8g

3. Grilled Salmon with Dill Sauce

Total Time: 30 minutes | Serves 2

Ingredients

- 2 (4-ounce) salmon fillets
- 1 tablespoon olive oil
- Salt and pepper to taste
- For the Dill Sauce:
- 1/4 cup plain Greek yogurt
- 1 tablespoon lemon juice
- 1 tablespoon chopped fresh dill
- 1 clove garlic, minced
- Salt and pepper to taste

Instructions

1. Preheat a grill or a grill pan to medium-high heat.
2. Brush the salmon fillets with olive oil and season with salt and pepper.
3. Grill the salmon for 4-6 minutes per side, or until cooked through.
4. In a small bowl, mix together the ingredients for the dill sauce.
5. Serve the grilled salmon with the dill sauce on the side.

Per serving: - Calories: 260 - Fiber: 0g - Carbs: 4g - Fat: 15g - Protein: 26g - Sugar: 2g

4. Turkey Meatballs in Marinara Sauce

Total Time: 40 minutes | Serves 2

Ingredients

- 1 lb ground turkey
- 1/4 cup breadcrumbs
- 1 egg, beaten
- 2 cloves garlic, minced
- 1 tablespoon chopped fresh parsley
- 1/2 teaspoon salt
- 1/4 teaspoon black pepper
- 1 cup marinara sauce
- 2 cups cooked whole wheat pasta

Instructions

1. Preheat your oven to 400°F.
2. In a mixing bowl, add the ground turkey, breadcrumbs, egg, garlic, parsley, salt, and pepper. Mix until well incorporated.
3. Roll the mixture into 12 meatballs, about 1-inch in size.
4. Place the meatballs on a baking sheet lined with parchment paper.
5. Bake for 15-20 minutes, or until the meatballs are cooked through.
6. In a saucepan, heat the marinara sauce over medium heat.
7. Add the cooked meatballs to the marinara sauce and simmer for 5 minutes.
8. Serve the meatballs and sauce over the cooked whole wheat pasta.

Per serving: - Calories: 350 - Fiber: 6g - Carbs: 35g - Fat: 12g - Protein: 32g - Sugar: 8g

5. Quinoa Stuffed Peppers

Total Time: 50 minutes | Serves 2

Ingredients

- 2 large bell peppers (halved and seeded)
- 1/2 cup cooked quinoa
- 1/2 cup diced tomatoes
- 1/4 cup diced onion
- 1 clove garlic, minced
- 1 tablespoon chopped fresh basil
- 1/4 teaspoon salt
- 1/8 teaspoon black pepper
- 1/4 cup shredded low-fat mozzarella cheese

Instructions

1. Preheat your oven to 375°F.
2. Place the bell pepper halves in a baking dish and set aside.
3. In a bowl, combine the cooked quinoa, diced tomatoes, onion, garlic, basil, salt, and pepper.
4. Spoon the quinoa mixture into the bell pepper halves.
5. Top the stuffed peppers with the shredded mozzarella cheese.
6. Bake for 25-30 minutes, or until the peppers are tender and the cheese is melted.

Per serving: - Calories: 180 - Fiber: 5g - Carbs: 24g - Fat: 5g - Protein: 12g - Sugar: 6g

6. Roasted Vegetable Medley

Total Time: 60 minutes | Serves 5

Ingredients

- 2 cups cubed butternut squash
- 1 cup sliced zucchini
- 1 cup sliced red bell pepper
- 1 cup sliced mushrooms
- 1 red onion (cut into wedges)
- 2 tablespoons olive oil
- 1 teaspoon dried thyme
- 1/2 teaspoon garlic powder
- 1/4 teaspoon salt
- 1/4 teaspoon black pepper

Instructions

1. Preheat your oven to 400°F (200°C).
2. In a large baking sheet, toss the cubed butternut squash, sliced zucchini, sliced red bell pepper, sliced mushrooms, and red onion wedges with olive oil, dried thyme, garlic powder, salt, and black pepper.
3. Roast for 35-40 minutes, stirring halfway, until the vegetables are tender and lightly browned.
4. Serve hot and enjoy.

Per serving: - Calories: 120 - Fiber: 4g - Carbs: 16g - Fats: 6g - Protein: 3g - Sugar: 6g

7. Garlic Shrimp Stir-Fry

Total Time: 40 minutes | Serves 5

Ingredients

- 1 lb. peeled and deveined shrimp
- 2 tablespoons olive oil
- 3 cloves garlic, minced
- 1 cup sliced mushrooms
- 1 cup snap peas
- 1 red bell pepper, sliced
- 2 tablespoons low-sodium soy sauce
- 1 teaspoon rice vinegar
- 1/4 teaspoon red pepper flakes (optional)
- Salt and black pepper to taste

Instructions

1. Heat the olive oil in a large skillet or wok over medium-high heat.
2. Add the minced garlic and sauté for 1 minute until fragrant.
3. Add the shrimp and cook for 2-3 minutes, stirring frequently, until the shrimp start to turn pink.
4. Add the sliced mushrooms, snap peas, and red bell pepper. Stir-fry for 5-7 minutes until the vegetables are tender-crisp.
5. Stir in the low-sodium soy sauce, rice vinegar, and red pepper flakes (optional). Season with salt and black pepper to taste.
6. Serve immediately over steamed brown rice or quinoa.

Per serving: - Calories: 160 - Fiber: 2g - Carbs: 6g - Fats: 6g - Protein: 21g - Sugar: 2g

8. Mushroom and Spinach Risotto

Total Time: 50 minutes | Serves 5

Ingredients

- 4 cups low-sodium vegetable broth
- 1 tablespoon olive oil
- 1 onion, diced
- 8 oz. sliced mushrooms
- 1 cup Arborio rice
- 1/2 cup dry white wine
- 2 cups fresh spinach, chopped
- 1/4 cup grated Parmesan cheese
- Salt and black pepper to taste

Instructions

1. In a saucepan, bring the vegetable broth to a simmer and keep it warm over low heat.
2. In a large skillet, heat the olive oil over medium heat. Add the diced onion and sauté for 3-4 minutes until translucent.
3. Add the sliced mushrooms and continue to sauté for 5 minutes.
4. Stir in the Arborio rice and coat it with the oil. Cook for 2-3 minutes, stirring constantly.
5. Pour in the white wine and stir until the wine is absorbed.
6. Ladle in the warm vegetable broth, 1/2 cup at a time, stirring continuously until the liquid is absorbed before adding more. Continue this process for 25-30 minutes, until the rice is tender and creamy.
7. Stir in the chopped fresh spinach and grated Parmesan cheese. Season with salt and black pepper to taste. Serve immediately and enjoy.

Per serving: - Calories: 230 - Fiber: 3g - Carbs: 34g - Fats: 6g - Protein: 9g - Sugar: 3g

9. Baked Cod with Herbs

Total Time: 30 minutes | Serves 5

Ingredients

- 1.5 lbs. cod fillets
- 2 tablespoons olive oil
- 2 tablespoons chopped fresh parsley
- 1 tablespoon chopped fresh thyme
- 1 tablespoon chopped fresh rosemary
- 1 teaspoon garlic powder
- 1/4 teaspoon salt
- 1/4 teaspoon black pepper

Instructions

1. Preheat your oven to 400°F (200°C).
2. Pat the cod fillets dry with paper towels and place them in a baking dish.
3. In a small bowl, mix together the olive oil, chopped fresh parsley, thyme, rosemary, garlic powder, salt, and black pepper.
4. Spread the herb mixture evenly over the top of the cod fillets.
5. Bake for 15-20 minutes, or until the cod is opaque and flakes easily with a fork.
6. Serve immediately and enjoy.

Per serving: - Calories: 160 - Fiber: 0g - Carbs: 0g - Fats: 6g - Protein: 25g - Sugar: 0g

10. Stuffed Acorn Squash with Quinoa and Cranberries

Total Time: 60 minutes | Serves 5

Ingredients

- 2 acorn squash (halved and seeded)
- 1 cup cooked quinoa
- 1/2 cup fresh cranberries
- 1/4 cup chopped walnuts
- 2 tablespoons maple syrup
- 1 teaspoon ground cinnamon
- 1/4 teaspoon salt
- 1/4 teaspoon black pepper

Instructions

1. Preheat your oven to 400°F (200°C).
2. Place the acorn squash halves, cut-side up, on a baking sheet. Roast for 30-40 minutes, or until the squash is tender when pierced with a fork.
3. In a medium bowl, combine the cooked quinoa, fresh cranberries, chopped walnuts, maple syrup, ground cinnamon, salt, and black pepper.
4. Scoop the quinoa mixture into the roasted acorn squash halves, dividing it evenly.
5. Return the stuffed squash to the oven and bake for an additional 15-20 minutes, or until the filling is heated through.
6. Serve hot and enjoy.

Per serving: - Calories: 190 - Fiber: 5g - Carbs: 30g - Fats: 7g - Protein: 5g - Sugar: 7g

11. Spaghetti Squash with Tomato Sauce

Total Time: 60 minutes | Serves 4

Ingredients

- 1 medium spaghetti squash (halved and seeded)
- 1 tbsp olive oil
- 1 onion, diced
- 3 garlic cloves, minced
- 1 (14 oz) can diced tomatoes
- 2 tbsp fresh basil, chopped
- 1 tsp dried oregano
- Salt and pepper to taste

Instructions

1. Preheat your oven to 400°F (200°C).
2. Place the spaghetti squash halves cut-side down on a baking sheet. Bake for 30-35 minutes, or until the squash is tender.
3. In a saucepan, heat the olive oil over medium heat. Add the onion and sauté for 5 minutes until translucent.
4. Add the garlic and sauté for 1 minute until fragrant.
5. Stir in the diced tomatoes, basil, and oregano. Season with salt and pepper.
6. Simmer the sauce for 10 minutes, stirring occasionally.
7. Use a fork to shred the spaghetti squash into strands.
8. Serve the spaghetti squash topped with the tomato sauce.

Per serving: - Calories: 120 - Fiber: 4g - Carbs: 18g - Fat: 5g - Protein: 3g - Sugar: 6g

12. Chicken and Vegetable Skewers

Total Time: 40 minutes | Serves 4

Ingredients

- 1 lb boneless, skinless chicken breasts, cubed
- 1 red bell pepper, (cut into 1-inch pieces)
- 1 zucchini, (cut into 1-inch pieces)
- 1 red onion, (cut into 1-inch pieces)
- 2 tbsp olive oil
- 1 tsp dried oregano
- 1 tsp paprika
- Salt and pepper to taste

Instructions

1. Preheat a grill or a grill pan to medium-high heat.
2. In a large bowl, toss the chicken, bell pepper, zucchini, and onion with the olive oil, oregano, paprika, salt, and pepper.
3. Thread the chicken and vegetables onto skewers, alternating the ingredients.
4. Grill the skewers for 12-15 minutes, turning occasionally, until the chicken is cooked through and the vegetables are tender.
5. Serve the skewers immediately.

Per serving: - Calories: 220 - Fiber: 3g - Carbs: 9g - Fat: 9g - Protein: 27g - Sugar: 5g

13. Pork Tenderloin with Mango Salsa

Total Time: 50 minutes | Serves 4

Ingredients

- 1 lb pork tenderloin
- 1 tbsp olive oil
- 1 mango, diced
- 1 red onion, diced
- 1 jalapeño (seeded and diced)
- 2 tbsp fresh cilantro, chopped
- Juice of 1 lime
- Salt and pepper to taste

Instructions

1. Preheat your oven to 400°F (200°C).
2. Season the pork tenderloin with salt and pepper.
3. In a large oven-safe skillet, heat the olive oil over medium-high heat. Sear the pork tenderloin on all sides, about 2-3 minutes per side.
4. Take the skillet to the oven and roast the pork for 20-25 minutes, or until it reaches an internal temperature of 145°F (63°C).
5. While the pork is roasting, prepare the mango salsa by combining the diced mango, red onion, jalapeño, cilantro, and lime juice in a bowl. Season with salt and pepper.
6. Let the pork rest for 5 minutes, then slice and serve with the mango salsa.

Per serving: - Calories: 230 - Fiber: 2g - Carbs: 14g - Fat: 8g - Protein: 26g - Sugar: 11g

14. Cauliflower Steak with Chimichurri Sauce

Total Time: 50 minutes | Serves 4

Ingredients

- 1 head of cauliflower (cut into 1-inch thick slices)
- 2 tbsp olive oil
- Salt and pepper to taste
- 1 cup fresh parsley, chopped
- 1/2 cup fresh cilantro, chopped
- 3 garlic cloves, minced
- 2 tbsp red wine vinegar
- 1/4 cup olive oil
- 1 tsp red pepper flakes (optional)

Instructions

1. Preheat your oven to 400°F (200°C).
2. Arrange the cauliflower slices on a baking sheet, brush with the 2 tbsp of olive oil, and season with salt and pepper.
3. Roast the cauliflower for 25-30 minutes, flipping halfway, until tender and lightly browned.
4. In a food processor, combine the parsley, cilantro, garlic, red wine vinegar, 1/4 cup olive oil, and red pepper flakes (optional). Pulse until well combined but still slightly chunky.
5. Serve the roasted cauliflower steaks topped with the chimichurri sauce.

Per serving: - Calories: 160 - Fiber: 5g - Carbs: 10g - Fat: 13g - Protein: 4g - Sugar: 4g

15. Turkey Chili with Beans

Total Time: 60 minutes | Serves 4

Ingredients

- 1 lb ground turkey
- 3 garlic cloves, minced
- 1 tsp ground cumin
- 1/4 tsp cayenne pepper (optional)
- 1 (15 oz) can diced tomatoes
- 1 (15 oz) can kidney beans (rinsed and drained)
- 1 (15 oz) can black beans (rinsed and drained)
- Salt and pepper to taste
- 1 onion, diced
- 2 tsp chili powder
- 1 tsp dried oregano

Instructions

1. In a large pot or Dutch oven, cook the ground turkey over medium-high heat, breaking it up with a wooden spoon, until browned, about 5-7 minutes.
2. Add the onion and garlic, and sauté for 3-4 minutes until the onion is translucent.
3. Stir in the chili powder, cumin, oregano, and cayenne pepper (optional). Cook for 1 minute to toast the spices.
4. Add the diced tomatoes, kidney beans, and black beans. Stir to combine.
5. Reduce the heat to medium-low and simmer the chili for 30-40 minutes, stirring occasionally, until the flavors have melded and the chili has thickened.
6. Season with salt and pepper to taste.
7. Serve the turkey chili hot, garnished with your desired toppings (avocado, cilantro, or low-fat sour cream).

Per serving: - Calories: 320 - Fiber: 11g - Carbs: 30g - Fat: 9g - Protein: 29g - Sugar: 6g

Snack Recipes

1. Almond and Date Energy Balls

Total Time: 15 minutes | Serves 2

Ingredients

- 1 cup (150g) raw almonds
- 1/2 cup (80g) pitted dates
- 2 tbsp (30ml) honey
- 1 tsp (5ml) vanilla extract
- 1/4 tsp (1.25ml) ground cinnamon

Instructions

1. In a food processor, blend the almonds until they form a coarse meal.
2. Add the pitted dates, honey, vanilla extract, and cinnamon. Blend until a sticky dough forms.
3. Scoop the mixture and roll into 12 equal-sized balls.
4. Store the energy balls in an airtight container in the refrigerator for up to 1 week.

Per serving: - Calories: 212 - Fiber: 4g - Carbs: 22g - Fats: 12g - Protein: 5g - Sugar: 16g

2. Cucumber and Hummus Bites

Total Time: 10 minutes | Serves 2

Ingredients

- 1 medium cucumber (sliced into 8 rounds)
- 1/2 cup (120g) hummus
- 2 tbsp (30ml) chopped fresh parsley (optional)

Instructions

1. Arrange the cucumber slices on a serving plate.
2. Top each cucumber slice with a spoonful of hummus.
3. Sprinkle with chopped fresh parsley (optional)

Per serving: - Calories: 75 - Fiber: 2g - Carbs: 8g - Fats: 4g - Protein: 3g - Sugar: 2g

3. Bell Pepper Strips with Guacamole

Total Time: 15 minutes | Serves 2

Ingredients

- 1 large ripe avocado (pitted and mashed)
- 2 tbsp (30ml) freshly squeezed lime juice
- 2 tbsp (30ml) finely chopped cilantro
- 1 garlic clove, minced
- 1/4 tsp (1.25ml) sea salt
- 2 medium bell peppers (cut into strips)

Instructions

1. In a bowl, add the mashed avocado, lime juice, cilantro, garlic, and sea salt. Mix well.
2. Arrange the bell pepper strips on a serving plate.
3. Serve the guacamole alongside the bell pepper strips for dipping.

Per serving: - Calories: 147 - Fiber: 7g - Carbs: 12g - Fats: 10g - Protein: 3g - Sugar: 5g

4. Mixed Berries with Whipped Cream

Total Time: 10 minutes | Serves 2

Ingredients

- 1 cup (150g) mixed berries (raspberries, blackberries, and blueberries)
- 1/2 cup (120ml) heavy whipping cream
- 1 tbsp (15ml) powdered sugar

Instructions

1. In a medium bowl, whip the heavy cream and powdered sugar until soft peaks form.
2. Divide the mixed berries into two serving bowls.
3. Top the berries with the whipped cream.

Per serving: - Calories: 165 - Fiber: 5g - Carbs: 15g - Fats: 11g - Protein: 2g - Sugar: 12g

5. Apricot and Almond Trail Mix

Total Time: 10 minutes | Serves 2

Ingredients

- 1/2 cup (75g) raw almonds
- 1/2 cup (80g) dried apricots, chopped
- 2 tbsp (30ml) unsweetened shredded coconut

Instructions

1. In a small bowl, combine the raw almonds, chopped dried apricots, and unsweetened shredded coconut.
2. Mix well and serve.

Per serving: - Calories: 187 - Fiber: 4g - Carbs: 16g - Fats: 13g - Protein: 5g - Sugar: 11g

6. Cherry Tomato Mozzarella Skewers

Total Time: 15 minutes | Serves 2

Ingredients

- 16 cherry tomatoes
- 8 small fresh mozzarella balls (or 1/2 cup (120g) cubed fresh mozzarella)
- 2 tbsp (30ml) balsamic glaze
- Fresh basil leaves (optional)

Instructions

1. Thread the cherry tomatoes and mozzarella balls onto 8 small skewers, alternating between the two.
2. Arrange the skewers on a serving platter.
3. Drizzle the balsamic glaze over the skewers.
4. Garnish with fresh basil leaves (optional)

Per serving: - Calories: 130 - Fiber: 1g - Carbs: 6g - Fats: 9g - Protein: 7g - Sugar: 5g

7. Carrot Sticks with Tzatziki Dip

Total Time: 20 minutes | Serves 2

Ingredients

- 1 cup (240g) plain Greek yogurt
- 1 cucumber (peeled, seeded, and grated)
- 2 tbsp (30ml) freshly squeezed lemon juice
- 1 garlic clove, minced
- 1 tsp (5ml) fresh dill, chopped
- 1/4 tsp (1.25ml) sea salt
- 4 medium carrots (peeled and cut into sticks)

Instructions

1. In a bowl, add the Greek yogurt, grated cucumber, lemon juice, garlic, fresh dill, and sea salt. Mix well to make the tzatziki dip.
2. Arrange the carrot sticks on a serving platter.
3. Serve the tzatziki dip alongside the carrot sticks for dipping.

Per serving: - Calories: 105 - Fiber: 3g - Carbs: 10g - Fats: 4g - Protein: 7g - Sugar: 6g

8. Hard-Boiled Eggs with Mustard

Total Time: 30 minutes | Serves 2

Ingredients

- 4 large eggs
- 2 tsp (10ml) Dijon mustard
- 1 tbsp (15ml) freshly squeezed lemon juice
- 1/4 tsp (1.25ml) sea salt
- 1/8 tsp (0.6ml) black pepper

Instructions

1. Place the eggs in a saucepan and cover with cold water by 1 inch (2.5 cm).
2. Bring the water to a boil over high heat, then remove from heat and cover. Let the eggs sit for 12 minutes.
3. Drain the hot water and cover the eggs with cold water. Let sit for 5 minutes.
4. Peel the eggs and place them in a bowl.
5. In a small bowl, mix the Dijon mustard, lemon juice, sea salt, and black pepper.
6. Drizzle the mustard mixture over the hard-boiled eggs and serve.

Per serving: - Calories: 140 - Fiber: 0g - Carbs: 2g - Fats: 10g - Protein: 12g - Sugar: 1g

9. Popcorn with Olive Oil and Herbs

Total Time: 20 minutes | Serves 2

Ingredients

- 1/4 cup (60ml) popcorn kernels
- 1 tbsp (15ml) olive oil
- 1 tsp (5ml) dried oregano
- 1/2 tsp (2.5ml) dried thyme
- 1/4 tsp (1.25ml) sea salt

Instructions

1. In a large saucepan with a lid, heat the popcorn kernels over medium heat, shaking the pan occasionally, until the popping slows to 2-3 seconds between pops.
2. Remove the pan from heat and immediately take the popped popcorn to a large bowl.
3. Drizzle the olive oil over the popcorn and sprinkle with the dried oregano, thyme, and sea salt.
4. Toss the popcorn to evenly coat with the oil and seasonings.

Per serving: - Calories: 130 - Fiber: 4g - Carbs: 14g - Fats: 7g - Protein: 3g - Sugar: 0g

10. Rice Cakes with Avocado and Cherry Tomatoes

Total Time: 20 minutes | Serves 2

Ingredients

- 4 whole grain rice cakes
- 1 ripe avocado, mashed
- 8 cherry tomatoes, halved
- 1 tbsp (15ml) fresh lemon juice
- 1/4 tsp (1.25ml) sea salt
- 1/8 tsp (0.6ml) black pepper

Instructions

1. Spread the mashed avocado evenly over the 4 rice cakes.
2. Top each rice cake with 4 cherry tomato halves.
3. Drizzle the lemon juice over the tomatoes and season with sea salt and black pepper.

Per serving: - Calories: 180 - Fiber: 7g - Carbs: 22g - Fats: 9g - Protein: 4g - Sugar: 2g

Dessert Recipes

1. Baked Peaches with Almond Crumble

Total Time: 50 minutes | Serves 3

Ingredients

- 3 medium peaches (halved and pitted)
- 2 tbsp rolled oats
- 2 tbsp almond flour
- 1 tbsp coconut sugar
- 1 tsp ground cinnamon
- 2 tbsp unsalted butter, softened

Instructions

1. Preheat your oven to 375°F.
2. Arrange peach halves in a baking dish.
3. In a small bowl, combine the oats, almond flour, coconut sugar, and cinnamon. Cut in the butter until the mixture is crumbly.
4. Spoon the crumble topping evenly over the peach halves.
5. Bake for 30-35 minutes, until the peaches are tender and the topping is lightly browned.
6. Serve warm and enjoy.

Per serving: - Calories: 160 - Fiber: 3g - Carbs: 21g - Fat: 9g - Protein: 2g - Sugar: 15g

2. Strawberry Frozen Yogurt

Total Time: 4 hours 20 minutes | Serves 3

Ingredients

- 2 cups fresh strawberries (hulled and sliced)
- 1 cup plain Greek yogurt
- 2 tbsp honey
- 1 tsp vanilla extract

Instructions

1. In a medium bowl, add the strawberries, yogurt, honey, and vanilla. Stir to mix well.
2. Pour the mixture into a shallow baking dish and freeze for 4 hours, stirring every 30 minutes, until frozen.
3. Scoop and serve immediately.

Per serving: - Calories: 130 - Fiber: 2g - Carbs: 18g - Fat: 4g - Protein: 8g - Sugar: 15g

3. Dark Chocolate-Dipped Strawberries

Total Time: 20 minutes | Serves 3

Ingredients

- 12 fresh strawberries
- 2 oz dark chocolate (70% cacao or higher), chopped

Instructions

1. Rinse the strawberries and pat them dry with a paper towel.
2. Melt the dark chocolate in a double boiler or in the microwave, stirring frequently until smooth.
3. Dip each strawberry into the melted chocolate, coating three-quarters of the berry.
4. Place the chocolate-dipped strawberries on a parchment-lined baking sheet and refrigerate for 10 minutes to set the chocolate.

Per serving: - Calories: 87 - Fiber: 2g - Carbs: 9g - Fat: 5g - Protein: 1g - Sugar: 7g

4. Pear and Walnut Crisp

Total Time: 50 minutes | Serves 3

Ingredients

- 3 medium pears (peeled, cored, and sliced)
- 2 tbsp lemon juice
- 1/4 cup old-fashioned oats
- 2 tbsp almond flour
- 1 tbsp coconut sugar
- 1/2 tsp ground cinnamon
- 2 tbsp unsalted butter, cubed

Instructions

1. Preheat your oven to 375°F.
2. In a bowl, toss the pear slices with lemon juice.
3. In a different bowl, combine the oats, almond flour, coconut sugar, and cinnamon. Cut in the butter until the mixture is crumbly.
4. Arrange the pear slices in a baking dish. Sprinkle the oat topping evenly over the top.
5. Bake for 30-35 minutes, until the pears are tender and the topping is lightly browned.
6. Serve warm and enjoy.

Per serving: - Calories: 170 - Fiber: 4g - Carbs: 24g - Fat: 8g - Protein: 2g - Sugar: 15g

5. Lemon Sorbet

Total Time: 5 hours | Serves 3

Ingredients

- 1 cup freshly squeezed lemon juice (about 5-6 lemons)
- 1/2 cup granulated sugar
- 1 cup water
- 1 tbsp lemon zest

Instructions

---

1. In a medium saucepan, combine the lemon juice, sugar, and water. Bring to a simmer, stirring occasionally, until the sugar has dissolved.
2. Remove from heat and stir in the lemon zest.
3. Pour the mixture into a shallow baking dish and freeze for 4 hours, stirring every 30 minutes, until frozen.
4. Scoop and serve immediately.

Per serving: - Calories: 120 - Fiber: 0g - Carbs: 30g - Fat: 0g - Protein: 0g - Sugar: 28g

6. Almond Flour Cookies

Total Time: 30 minutes | Serves 2

Ingredients

- 1 cup almond flour
- 2 tbsp coconut sugar
- 1/4 tsp baking soda
- 1/4 tsp ground cinnamon
- 2 tbsp coconut oil, melted
- 1 tsp vanilla extract

Instructions

1. Preheat your oven to 350°F. Line a baking sheet with parchment paper.
2. In a medium bowl, whisk together the almond flour, coconut sugar, baking soda, and cinnamon.
3. Add the melted coconut oil and vanilla extract, and mix until a dough forms.
4. Scoop out 2-tbsp portions of the dough and place them on the baking sheet, spacing them about 2 inches apart.
5. Bake for 12-15 minutes, until lightly golden. Allow to cool on the baking sheet for 5 minutes before taking to a wire rack.

Per serving: - Calories: 175 - Fiber: 2g - Carbs: 12g - Fat: 15g - Protein: 4g - Sugar: 8g

7. Poached Pears in Red Wine

Total Time: 50 minutes | Serves 2

Ingredients

- 2 pears (peeled, halved, and cored)
- 1 cup red wine
- 1/4 cup honey
- 1 cinnamon stick
- 2 whole cloves
- 1 strip of lemon zest

Instructions

1. In a medium saucepan, combine the red wine, honey, cinnamon stick, cloves, and lemon zest. Bring to a simmer over medium heat.
2. Add the pear halves to the saucepan, making sure they are submerged in the liquid. Reduce heat to low and simmer for 20-25 minutes, or until the pears are tender when pierced with a fork.
3. Using a slotted spoon, transfer the pear halves to a serving dish.
4. Increase the heat to medium-high and let the poaching liquid simmer for 5-7 minutes, until it has reduced by about half and thickened slightly.
5. Pour the warm poaching liquid over the pears and serve.

Per serving: - Calories: 180 - Fiber: 3g - Carbs: 28g - Fat: 0g - Protein: 1g - Sugar: 22g

8. Greek Yogurt Parfait with Fresh Berries

Total Time: 15 minutes | Serves 2

Ingredients

- 1 cup plain Greek yogurt
- 1 cup mixed fresh berries (blueberries, raspberries, and blackberries)
- 2 tbsp honey

Instructions

1. In two parfait glasses or bowls, layer half of the Greek yogurt, followed by half of the fresh berries, and drizzle with 1 tbsp of honey.
2. Repeat the layers with the remaining yogurt, berries, and honey.
3. Serve immediately and enjoy.

Per serving: - Calories: 150 - Fiber: 3g - Carbs: 20g - Fat: 5g - Protein: 12g - Sugar: 17g

9. Mango Sorbet

Total Time: 4 hours | Serves 2

Ingredients

- 2 cups diced ripe mango
- 1/4 cup water
- 2 tbsp lime juice
- 1 tbsp honey

Instructions

1. In a blender, combine the mango, water, lime juice, and honey. Blend until smooth.
2. Pour the mango mixture into a shallow baking dish and place in the freezer. Stir the mixture every 30 minutes for the first 2 hours, then every hour until completely frozen, about 4 hours total.
3. Scoop the frozen sorbet into bowls and serve immediately.

Per serving: - Calories: 110 - Fiber: 2g - Carbs: 27g - Fat: 0g - Protein: 1g - Sugar: 24g

10. Pistachio Date Balls

Total Time: 25 minutes | Serves 2

Ingredients

- 1 cup shelled pistachios
- 1 cup pitted dates
- 1 tbsp honey
- 1 tsp vanilla extract
- Pinch of sea salt

Instructions

1. In a food processor, pulse the pistachios until they are finely chopped but not a powder.
2. Add the dates, honey, vanilla, and salt to the food processor and blend until the mixture forms a sticky, cohesive dough.
3. Scoop out tablespoon-sized portions of the dough and roll them into balls.
4. Place the pistachio date balls on a parchment-lined plate or baking sheet and refrigerate for at least 10 minutes before serving.

Per serving: - Calories: 180 - Fiber: 4g - Carbs: 25g - Fat: 9g - Protein: 4g - Sugar: 19g

Beverages

---

1. Cucumber Mint Infused Water

Prep Time: 10 minutes | Refrigerating Time: 30 minutes | Serves 2

Ingredients

- 4 cups filtered water
- 1 cucumber, sliced
- 6-8 fresh mint leaves

Instructions

1. In a pitcher, combine the water, cucumber slices, and mint leaves.
2. Refrigerate for at least 30 minutes to allow the flavors to infuse.
3. Serve chilled and enjoy.

Per serving: - Calories: 8 - Fiber: 0.5g - Carbs: 2g - Fats: 0g - Protein: 0g - Sugar: 1g

2. Ginger Turmeric Tea

Total Time: 20 minutes | Serves 2

Ingredients

- 2 cups filtered water
- 1-inch piece of fresh ginger (peeled and sliced)
- 1 teaspoon ground turmeric
- 1 tablespoon honey (optional)
- Squeeze of lemon juice (optional)

Instructions

1. In a small saucepan, bring the water to a boil.
2. Add the ginger slices and turmeric. Reduce heat and simmer for 5-7 minutes.
3. Strain the tea into mugs.
4. Stir in honey and lemon juice (optional).
5. Serve hot and enjoy.

Per serving: - Calories: 30 - Fiber: 0g - Carbs: 8g - Fats: 0g - Protein: 0g - Sugar: 7g

3. Lemon Balm Iced Tea

Prep Time: 20 minutes | Refrigerating Time: 2 hours | Serves 2

Ingredients

- 4 cups filtered water
- 6-8 fresh lemon balm leaves
- 2 tablespoons honey (optional)

Instructions

1. In a small saucepan, bring the water to a boil.
2. Remove from the heat and add the lemon balm leaves. Cover and let steep for 10 minutes.
3. Strain the tea into a pitcher and stir in honey (optional).
4. Refrigerate until chilled, at least 2 hours.
5. Serve over ice.

Per serving: - Calories: 30 - Fiber: 0g - Carbs: 8g - Fats: 0g - Protein: 0g - Sugar: 7g

4. Watermelon Basil Cooler

Total Time: 15 minutes | Serves 2

Ingredients

- 2 cups diced seedless watermelon
- 1/4 cup fresh basil leaves
- 1 tablespoon lime juice
- 1 cup sparkling water

Instructions

1. In a blender, add the diced watermelon, basil leaves, and lime juice. Blend until smooth.
2. Pour the watermelon mixture into two glasses.
3. Top each glass with 1/2 cup of sparkling water.
4. Serve immediately and enjoy.

Per serving: - Calories: 45 - Fiber: 1g - Carbs: 11g - Fats: 0g - Protein: 1g - Sugar: 9g

5. Watermelon Mint Agua Fresca

Total Time: 15 minutes | Serves 2

Ingredients

- 2 cups diced seedless watermelon
- 1/4 cup fresh mint leaves
- 1 tablespoon lime juice
- 1 cup filtered water
- Ice

Instructions

1. In a blender, add the watermelon, mint leaves, and lime juice. Blend until smooth.
2. Pour the watermelon mixture into a pitcher and stir in the water.
3. Serve over ice.

Per serving: - Calories: 35 - Fiber: 1g - Carbs: 9g - Fats: 0g - Protein: 1g - Sugar: 7g

6. Blueberry Lavender Lemonade

Total Time: 15 minutes | Serves 2

Ingredients

- 1 cup fresh or frozen blueberries
- 2 tablespoons dried lavender flowers
- 1/4 cup fresh lemon juice
- 2 tablespoons honey
- 1 cup cold water
- Ice

Instructions

1. In a small saucepan, combine the blueberries, lavender, lemon juice, and honey. Bring to a simmer and cook for 5 minutes, stirring occasionally.
2. Strain the mixture through a fine-mesh sieve, pressing on the solids to extract as much liquid as possible.
3. In a pitcher, combine the strained blueberry-lavender syrup and cold water. Stir to combine.
4. Serve over ice and enjoy.

Per serving: - Calories: 60 - Fiber: 2g - Carbs: 16g - Fats: 0g - Protein: 0g - Sugar: 13g

7. Hibiscus Ginger Kombucha

Prep Time: 15 minutes | Fermentation Time: 1 to 2 days | Serves 2

Ingredients

- 4 cups brewed hibiscus tea, cooled
- 1 tablespoon grated fresh ginger
- 1 cup unflavored kombucha
- 1 tablespoon honey (optional)

Instructions

1. In a large jar or pitcher, combine the cooled hibiscus tea and grated ginger.
2. Add the kombucha and stir gently to combine.
3. Cover the jar with a cloth or coffee filter and secure it with a rubber band.
4. Allow the mixture to ferment at room temperature for 24-48 hours.
5. Strain the kombucha through a fine-mesh sieve, discarding the ginger.
6. Stir in honey (optional) and serve chilled.

Per serving: - Calories: 40 - Fiber: 0g - Carbs: 9g - Fats: 0g - Protein: 0g - Sugar: 6g

8. Pineapple Cilantro Limeade

Total Time: 15 minutes | Serves 2

Ingredients

- 1 cup diced pineapple
- 1/4 cup fresh cilantro leaves
- 2 tablespoons fresh lime juice
- 1 cup cold water
- Ice

Instructions

1. In a blender, add the diced pineapple, cilantro leaves, and lime juice. Blend until smooth.
2. Pour the pineapple-cilantro mixture into a pitcher and stir in the cold water.
3. Serve over ice and enjoy.

Per serving: - Calories: 40 - Fiber: 1g - Carbs: 10g - Fats: 0g - Protein: 0g - Sugar: 8g

9. Rosemary Grapefruit Sparkler

Prep Time: 10 minutes | Refrigerating Time: 30 minutes | Serves 2

Ingredients

- 1 cup freshly squeezed grapefruit juice
- 2 sprigs fresh rosemary
- 1 cup sparkling water
- Ice

Instructions

1. In a pitcher, combine the grapefruit juice and rosemary sprigs.
2. Refrigerate for at least 30 minutes to allow the flavors to infuse.
3. Remove the rosemary sprigs and stir in the sparkling water.
4. Serve over ice and enjoy.

Per serving: - Calories: 50 - Fiber: 0g - Carbs: 12g - Fats: 0g - Protein: 1g - Sugar: 10g

10. Blackberry Sage Sparkling Water

Total Time: 15 minutes | Serves 2

Ingredients

- 1 cup fresh blackberries
- 6-8 fresh sage leaves
- 1 cup sparkling water
- Ice

Instructions

1. In a small saucepan, gently muddle the blackberries and sage leaves.
2. Cook over medium heat for 3-4 minutes, stirring occasionally, until the blackberries release their juices.
3. Strain the blackberry-sage mixture through a fine-mesh sieve, pressing on the solids to extract as much liquid as possible.
4. In a pitcher, combine the strained blackberry-sage syrup and sparkling water. Stir to combine.
5. Serve over ice and enjoy.

Per serving: - Calories: 30 - Fiber: 2g - Carbs: 7g - Fats: 0g - Protein: 0g - Sugar: 5g

Conclusion

Congratulations for taking the first step towards controlling your gout with a nutritious, low-purine diet! By following the tasty recipes and meal plan in this cookbook, you'll lay the groundwork for long-term success in managing your gout symptoms and improving your overall health.

Remember that controlling gout is a continuing process, not a fast cure. The idea is to make long-term adjustments to your diet and lifestyle. Continue experimenting with the low-purine foods you've learned about in this book, and don't be afraid to vary things up to make your meals interesting and fulfilling.

As you go ahead, keep an eye on your uric acid levels and gout flare-ups. Pay attention to how your body reacts to various meals and make modifications as necessary. Don't be afraid to check with your healthcare provider or a trained dietitian to verify you're on the correct road.

In addition to food, be sure to integrate regular exercise into your regimen. Walking, swimming, and low-impact yoga are all good ways to decrease inflammation and enhance joint health.

Remember, you are not alone on this path. Reach out to support groups, both online and in your town, to connect with individuals who understand the difficulties of living with gout. Sharing your experiences and advice may be very empowering and inspirational.

With perseverance, patience, and a dedication to your health, you may regain control of your gout and live a pain-free lifestyle. I wish you the best as you continue to nurture your body and mind with the benefits of a gout-friendly diet.

2-Week Meal Plan

WEEK 1

	BREAKFAST	LUNCH	DINNER	SNACK/DESSERT
DAY 1	CINNAMON RAISIN TOAST WITH RICOTTA	CHICKPEA AND CUCUMBER SALAD	QUINOA STUFFED PEPPERS	LEMON SORBET
DAY 2	COTTAGE CHEESE WITH PINEAPPLE	EGGPLANT AND TOMATO PANINI	MUSHROOM AND SPINACH RISOTTO	PISTACHIO DATE BALLS
DAY 3	ALMOND BUTTER TOAST WITH SLICED APPLES	MUSHROOM BARLEY SOUP	CHICKEN AND VEGETABLE SKEWERS	HARD-BOILED EGGS WITH MUSTARD
DAY 4	BANANA WALNUT SMOOTHIE	CAPRESE SALAD WITH BALSAMIC GLAZE	LENTIL AND VEGETABLE STEW	PEAR AND WALNUT CRISP
DAY 5	BREAKFAST BURRITO WITH BLACK BEANS	TURKEY AND SPINACH ROLL-UPS	GARLIC SHRIMP STIR-FRY	CARROT STICKS WITH TZATZIKI DIP
DAY 6	WHOLE GRAIN PANCAKES WITH MAPLE SYRUP	SHRIMP AND AVOCADO SALAD	SPAGHETTI SQUASH WITH TOMATO SAUCE	CUCUMBER AND HUMMUS BITES
DAY 7	FRUIT SALAD WITH MINT	SALMON AND ASPARAGUS FOIL PACKETS	CAULIFLOWER STEAK WITH CHIMICHURRI SAUCE	RICE CAKES WITH AVOCADO AND CHERRY TOMATOES

WEEK 2 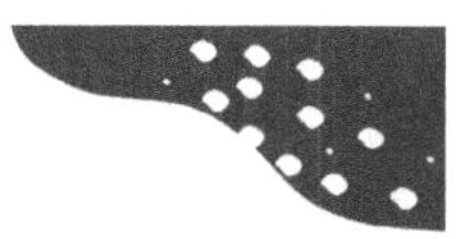

	BREAKFAST	LUNCH	DINNER	SNACK/DESSERT
DAY 1	GREEN SMOOTHIE WITH KALE AND PINEAPPLE	LENTIL SALAD WITH CHERRY TOMATOES	TURKEY MEATBALLS IN MARINARA SAUCE	DARK CHOCOLATE-DIPPED STRAWBERRIES
DAY 2	MUESLI WITH ALMOND MILK	ZUCCHINI NOODLES WITH PESTO	ROASTED VEGETABLE MEDLEY	APRICOT AND ALMOND TRAIL MIX
DAY 3	SCRAMBLED EGGS WITH SPINACH	EGG SALAD SANDWICH ON WHOLE WHEAT BREAD	GRILLED SALMON WITH DILL SAUCE	MIXED BERRIES WITH WHIPPED CREAM
DAY 4	BUCKWHEAT PORRIDGE WITH CINNAMON	SPINACH AND GOAT CHEESE STUFFED CHICKEN BREAST	STUFFED ACORN SQUASH WITH QUINOA AND CRANBERRIES	ALMOND AND DATE ENERGY BALLS
DAY 5	AVOCADO TOAST WITH TOMATO SLICES	ROASTED BEET AND GOAT CHEESE SALAD	TURKEY CHILI WITH BEANS	POPCORN WITH OLIVE OIL AND HERBS
DAY 6	TOMATO BASIL BRUSCHETTA	TURKEY AND AVOCADO WRAP	PORK TENDERLOIN WITH MANGO SALSA	BAKED PEACHES WITH ALMOND CRUMBLE
DAY 7	SMOKED SALMON AND CREAM CHEESE BAGEL	GRILLED CHICKEN CAESAR SALAD	BAKED HALIBUT WITH ASPARAGUS	POACHED PEARS IN RED WINE